The No B.S. Diet

Science-Based Recommendations to Stay Healthy and Medication Free—
Without the B.S.

By

JOEL KAHN, MD, FACC
Founder, Kahn Center for Cardiac Longevity
Clinical Professor of Medicine and Cardiology
Wayne State University School of Medicine

I have known Dr. Kahn for many years, and he has always been an inspiring and innovative leader in our field, as well as being a knowledgeable and compassionate doctor. His current goal to prevent one million heart attacks by early detection and lifestyle education is just what this country needs as it suffers from so many chronic diseases. By focusing on prevention with lifestyle, our future will be filled with healthier aging, making for more productive and enjoyable lives. Congratulations to Dr. Kahn for taking this on!

Kim Allan Williams, Sr., M.D., FACC, FAHA, FASNC
President, American College of Cardiology
James B. Herrick Professor
Chief, Division of Cardiology
Rush University Medical Center

Dr. Kahn is the rare physician who practices both state-of-the-art cardiac care, including interventional therapies, combined with advanced training in nutrition. His lectures and his writings, and his clinical benefits in treating his patients with plant-based, whole-foods diets have inspired many and placed him as a leader in lifestyle medicine. To top it off: his precepts and practices are congruous: he practices what he preaches. All of this makes him a model for the physician of the future.

Hans Diehl, DrHsc, MPH, FACN
Founder of the Lifestyle Medicine Institute and the Complete Health Improvement Program Clinical. Professor of Preventive Medicine, Loma Linda University, School of Medicine

This publication contains the opinion of the author. It is intended to provide helpful and informative material on the subject matters covered. It is sold with the understanding that the author and publisher are not engaged in rendering medical or other professional services in this report. If the reader requires personal medical health assistance or advice, a competent professional should be consulted.

The author and publisher specifically disclaim any responsibility for any liability, loss or risk, personal or otherwise, which is incurred as a consequence, directly or indirectly, of the use and application of any of the contents of this report.

Cover photograph: © Monni Must

Table of Contents

Dr. Joel Kahn: Professional Biography

Dr. Joel Kahn is a cardiologist on a personal mission to prevent one million heart attacks over the next two years. The US Department Health and Human Services and the Surgeon General embrace this goal of 1 Million Heart Attacks Prevented.

Dr. Kahn graduated summa cum laude from the University of Michigan, Ann Arbor, and practices a brand of cardiology combining the best of Western and complimentary therapies for total healing.

Known as "America's Holistic Heart Doc," Dr. Kahn has been practicing invasive, interventional and preventive cardiology in Detroit since 1990. He is a Clinical Professor of Medicine (Cardiology) at Wayne State University School of Medicine and Associate Professor of Medicine at Oakland University Beaumont School of Medicine.

In 2013, Dr. Kahn received a certification from the University of South Florida in Metabolic Cardiology and became the first physician in the world to complete the program. The American Academy of Anti-Aging Medicine has also certified Dr. Kahn in Metabolic Cardiology.

Over the past 25 years, Dr. Kahn has improved the lives and vitality of thousands of his patients, taking many of them from chronic health limitations to vibrant living. His devotion to patient care has earned him top honors, and he has been nominated as a Top Doctor in Cardiology for many years straight.

Dr. Kahn's patients and peer doctors recognize his passion for education and prevention.

Reader's Digest magazine selected Dr. Kahn for their Holistic Heart Doc column, and their publishing arm published his book, *The Whole Heart Solution,* a #1 Top Selling book. His second book, *Dead Execs Don't Get Bonuses* was published in 2015 and is on the #1 Bestseller List as well.

The Huffington Post and MindBodyGreen.com publish Dr. Kahn's medical views for a combined circulation 50.1 million unique monthly visitors. He frequently appears as a guest on radio, TV and podcasts. Dr. Kahn also appears regularly on Fox 2 TV in Detroit as a health commentator. He is also a member of the Yahoo Health Advisory Board, and he sits on The Food Babe Advisory Council.

To learn more about Dr. Kahn, visit www.drjoelkahn.com.

Introduction: None of the B.S.

I am still amazed by the science of the power of food as information. After training for years to treat heart attacks with balloons and stents, *I learned that food combined with simple lifestyle measures can actually prevent heart attacks and blockages*.

How could I not follow this path and teach my patients the same?

I have been doing just that for 25 years and feel great every day. I want to help you too. I decided long ago to eat a diet consisting of vegetables, fruits, whole grains and to avoid all animal and dairy products as a key step to better my health.

My family has made the same decision as well.

You do not have to adopt my personal diet as yours, but I do want you to know the reasons I made my choices. I also want you to know why I teach them to my patients and to others worldwide via my public speaking, articles and YouTube videos.

I am a proud founding member of the Plant-Based Nutrition Support Group (www.pbnsg.org), a group of nearly 1,500 members who meet monthly to discuss practical ways to enhance personal health and vitality.

The group embraces people from every walk of life: factory workers, accountants, lawyers, teachers, police and firemen and retired people. Within the group, each and every person has seen with their own eyes and felt within their bodies how dietary changes can make a huge difference in their health.

Nevertheless, this is not an all-or-nothing proposition.

You decide what makes sense to you and what you are willing to do. Each and every incremental change will make a difference in your health, vitality and life's enjoyments.

What's All the Fuss About?

Science establishes some basic truths about what to eat for health. So why are people constantly jumping from one food plan to another?

One possible explanation: the media highlights a study that says, "Eat this—and avoid that." Or they highlight the latest craze, fad diet or trendy doctor.

Following the hot trends can seem so confusing. Have we lost our minds and allowed ourselves to be yanked this way or that way when it comes to eating?

Do we no longer know how to eat? A new plan, a new miracle diet, new data pops up seemingly every five minutes.

I promise you this: I follow the medical literature carefully for my own health and that of my family in order to advise my patients and to enhance my roles as a speaker and professor of medicine and cardiology.

My conclusion? We have actually lost our path as we drift from one new fad to another.

So much B.S.!

As a student of nutrition and a graduate the University of South Florida with an advanced degree in Metabolic Cardiology, I sense utter confusion in my patients, my family and even amongst other medical professionals.

Butter, bacon, beef, kale, fruit, fats, carbs, protein… Which are good? Which are bad?

Medical literature provides answers that are often hidden by special interests or Big Food lobbies that blur the truths.

So much B.S.!

So I give you this, short and sweet: The No B.S. Diet.

Simple rules and lessons from science. I wrote it so you can read it in 30 minutes or an hour—and use the knowledge for a lifetime.

To health, happiness and clarity. And no B.S.!

Dr. Joel Kahn

Part I: Food Lessons from the Science Without the B.S.

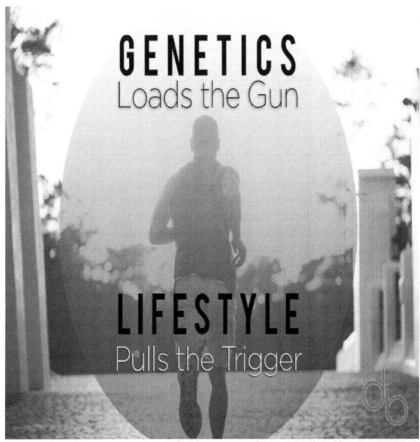

(Graphic courtesy of Doctor Bart http://bartprecourt.com/)

If You Only Have 10 Minutes – Important Nutrition Lessons

If your lifestyle is good, your genes get the message to make good proteins that promote health. In fact, cancer and heart genes shift from responding unhealthily to healthily within weeks of a clean, plant-strong diet.

Within less than an hour of eating a high-fat meal like an Egg McMuffin, your arteries show a major drop in health. Fast food, like the Egg McMuffin and similar products, can be poison and should be skipped.

Eating whole grains like whole wheat breads and pasta directly results in less heart disease, diabetes, cancer and obesity. Eating these foods is wise unless you have celiac disease.

Eating soybean products like edamame, tempeh or organic tofu produces less heart disease, less cancer and longer lifespans. Soy can be a joy.

Raw nuts and seeds give rise to longer lives and less heart disease, diabetes and obesity. If you are not allergic, a small handful can be healthy.

Colorful fruits and vegetables contain chemicals called polyphenols that lower your cholesterol and strengthen your arteries. Eat a rainbow of colorful produce.

Meat, including fish, directly connects you to developing a wide array of health problems. The worst offenders? Processed meats like hot dogs and bologna. Cut out or cut back the amount of meat you eat. Begin slowly by eliminating meat one day a week by starting Meatless Mondays.

While you cut back on meat, increase your servings of whole fruits and vegetables. Make a habit of eating five or more servings daily and you will reduce your risk of a heart attack.

A country of five million did it, and so can you. Finland's high heart attack rate dropped over 80 percent by reducing animal fats in the diet. They cut back on butter—and better health followed. See if you can cut back on butter and animal fats, too.

Cut back on salt, a health offender that can raise your blood pressure and damage your arteries. Be on the lookout for hidden salt in bread, pizza, canned soups and poultry, including chicken.

Which damages health first: the chicken or the egg? When healthy people eat whole eggs, their cholesterol goes up. So does the amount of plaque in their arteries! Know this: all animal products contain cholesterol and saturated fats.

If You Only Have 10 Minutes – Important Nutrition Lessons *(Cont'd)*

Just like adding a colorful variety of fruits and vegetables to your diet, adding a colorful array of spices like cinnamon, nutmeg, parsley, turmeric, rosemary, cloves and ginger can be the quickest way to boosting the nutritional values of any meal. Use spices regularly.

One final note about food preparation: When you BBQ on the grill, a chemical process occurs that can literally age you fast. Avoid grilling dry food. Use marinades, including black beer, at lower temperatures or bake or steam instead of grilling.

Lesson: My Family History is So Bad, Why Bother with All This?

Blaming it all on your family, no disrespect, is B.S. When people tell me that heart disease runs in the family, I say, "That is because *no one runs* in the family."

Birds of a feather flock together, and families eating the same processed diet, sitting in front of the same TVs and smoking the same Marlboro cigarettes get the same diseases. This is NOT genetic predisposition—but a lifestyle choice.

The No B.S. Diet is based on the fact that genes play a role—but only a small role—in overall health. Experts, including Dr. Sanjay Gupta, Chief Medical Correspondent for CNN, view genetics as contributing to 20 to 30 percent of chronic diseases like heart disease, leaving 70 to 80 percent to lifestyle.

In fact, if your lifestyle is good, your genes get the message to play nice and make good proteins, thus promoting health.

Further, science has shown that:

- Within three months, men with prostate cancer who begin a healthy lifestyle program turn off genes that cause cancer and turn on genes that fight cancer. Hundreds of them. Your fork can be like powerful chemotherapy with none of the side effects. Of course, always consult with your health team before making any changes to your medical protocols.
- Within three months of adopting a healthy lifestyle, patients with heart disease turned on genes that fight inflammation and artery damage and turned off genes that cause damage. Again, your fork can be like a potent medicine with none of the side effects.
- Within three months of changing to a healthy diet and lifestyle, genes that cause aging slow down and an enzyme called telomerase turns on to reverse aging. The real fountain of youth is filled with green tea and filtered water to bathe your body in health.

So if someone tells you it is too late to change your health by changing your diet, just say: "That is B.S."

For more information, read my article called "How The Food You Eat Changes Your Genes" at www.mindbodygreen.com.

Lesson: Food is Information, Not B.S.

Did you learn in school that food can speak to your arteries, your genes, even your brain? You probably know that if you eat French fries and ice cream day after day you are more likely to feel crappy, have low energy, struggle with poor mental focus, suffer from a sick stomach and get poor sleep.

Did you know these foods can make you sick enough to result in dying prematurely? These and other foods can provide crucial information to your body within an hour or less.

Let me share with you one important experiment. Have you ever eaten an Egg McMuffin? Researchers at the University of Maryland fed one of these to volunteers on one day—the high fat meal—and a low fat meal on another day.

What happened to their arteries an hour later?

Nothing bad happened to the arteries of those who ate the low fat meal. On the other hand, those who ate the high fat meal experienced fast, powerful and harmful effects to their arteries that lasted for almost seven hours.

Just eating one Egg McMuffin was like a bomb going off in their arteries. Poison. Not B.S.!

Stay away from fast food! It causes fast harm that sticks around.

To learn more, my article entitled "Is Your Breakfast Killing You?" may help at www.mindbodygreen.com/0-8138/is-your-breakfast-killing-you.html.

Lesson: Whole Grains Are Healthy, Not B.S.

The idea that grains, including whole grains, should be avoided routinely surfaces in the media and spreads far and wide. This happens despite the fact that the Harvard School of Public Health advises that 25 percent of your plate should be full of whole grains like whole wheat, brown rice and whole-grain pasta.

What is the No B.S. science about grains?
- Whole grains lower heart risk. A study of more than 400,000 participants found that the highest consumption of whole grains reduced the risk of heart-related issues by about 25 percent.
- Whole grains lower diabetes risk. A study showed that the more whole grains consumed, the lower the risk of type 2 diabetes mellitus.
- Whole grains reduce cancer risk. Colorectal cancer remains a major cause of death in the Western world, and evidence shows that whole grains may be preventive. Data from 25 studies indicate that three servings of whole grains a day reduced cancer risk by almost 20 percent. Evidence shows that fiber from legumes is beneficial, and eating them can lower cancer risk by almost 40 percent.
- Whole grains prevent obesity. Studies in 2010 connected whole grain consumption and body weight, only to discover that increased whole grain intake was modestly associated with lower body weight.
- Whole grains promote a long life. A study analyzing the amount of whole grains eaten by more than 360,000 people found that the more grains participants ate, the longer they lived.

The No B.S. solution?
If you do not have celiac disease and if eating whole grains does not upset your stomach, eat a lot of them and enjoy the benefits of the fiber, the vitamins and the minerals.
This is not about eating cakes, cookies or donuts but WHOLE grains. No B.S.!

<u>Lesson: Whole Grains Are Healthy, Not B.S.</u> (*Cont'd*)

If you want to learn more, you can read my article entitled "5 Reasons Grains Aren't As Bad As Everyone Says" at <u>www.mindbodygreen.com/0-18252/5-reasons-grains-arent-as-bad-as-everyone-says.html</u>.

Lesson: Soy Can Be a Joy

Following whole grains, few foods suffer from as bad a reputation as soy.

I know that a big block of tofu, however healthy, offers little to no appeal. But if you learn to buy organic tofu, edamame, soy milk or tempeh (fermented soy, all available in stores), you can make smart, delicious moves by adding these into salads, stir fries and casseroles.

Beware of soy isolates found in many food bars, which I personally avoid.

Let's explore the No B.S. science on soy:

- <u>Soy and Heart Attacks.</u> A study comparing 1,312 cases of first-time heart attack sufferers with 2,235 control subjects found that an unhealthy dietary pattern increased the risk of heart attack; whereas, an increased intake of vegetables, fruits and tofu led to a significant drop in heart attack rates.
- <u>Soy and Prostate Cancer</u>. A large study found that regular consumption of soy halved the risk of this serious disease.
- <u>Soy and Breast Cancer</u>. Japanese scientists identified studies that showed everything from a slight to a significant reduction in breast cancer with increased intake of soy foods.
- <u>Soy and Ovarian Cancer</u>. In southern China, regular soy intake resulted in dramatically lower rates of ovarian cancer. The more soy the women ate, the lower their risk of this type of cancer.
- <u>Soy and Mortality</u>. The Singapore Chinese Health Study examined more than 52,000 men and women free of chronic diseases. Up to a 25 percent less risk of death during the study period—and fewer heart-disease and cancer deaths—stemmed from a pattern of eating a vegetable, fruit and soy-rich diet.

If you want more details, read my article entitled "Why Soy Isn't As Bad For You As Everyone Says" at www.mindbodygreen.com/0-17741/why-soy-isnt-as-bad-for-you-as-everyone-says.html.

Lesson: Nuts and Seeds for Health

Nuts have a mixed reputation as a healthy food. Partly to blame is the rise in serious allergies. The fact that so many packaged nuts have added salt, sugar and oils taints the reputation of these wholesome provisions.

Let's see what raw nuts and seeds can do for you:

- Nuts can help with weight control. People incorporating any nuts into their diet were less likely to deal with obesity and metabolic syndrome, as determined in the Adventist Health Study. Other studies showed that eating nuts does not lead to weight gain.
- Nuts may reduce heart deaths in the elderly. In the Adventist Health Study examining death in residents over age 84 years old, those who ate nuts more than five times a week reduced their risk of overall death by nearly 20 percent. Of the same group, heart disease deaths decreased by a stunning 40 percent.
- Walnuts can lower cholesterol. In a small study comparing those eating a walnut-rich diet to a control group over eight weeks, the walnut diet participants' total cholesterol was reduced.
- Ground flaxseed lowers blood pressure. In an amazing six-month study, people eating 30 grams of milled flaxseed daily reduced systolic and diastolic blood pressure comparable to taking a prescription medication to reduce blood pressure.
- Chia seeds improve markers of diabetes, inflammation and body weight. Raw nuts, even peanuts, free of added salt, sugar and oil, can be a grab-and-go energy boost that helps your health. They are rich in calories, so a handful a day is about the limit.

If you want to learn more, read the article I wrote entitled "10 Reasons To Eat Way More Nuts & Seeds" at www.mindbodygreen.com/0-17256/10-reasons-to-eat-way-more-nuts-seeds.html.

Lesson: Why Colorful Foods Power Your Health (Not Skittles!)

Why are colorful fruits and vegetables so healthy? Why do blueberries lower your blood pressure and make your arteries younger?

Blueberries' secret: they possess chemicals that can heal your body. Blueberries are a rich source of polyphenols. When you eat polyphenols, your health skyrockets.

One broad type of polyphenols is found in red fruits, black radishes, onions, coffees, cereals and spices. Another type of polyphenol is found in foods such as soy, berries, herbs, broccoli, tomatoes, citrus fruits and juices and tea. Additionally, wine, nuts and flaxseed can contribute more polyphenols to your diet.

Polyphenols improve your health in six ways. They do all of the following:

1. Lower your cholesterol;
2. Lower your blood pressure;
3. Improve your artery function;
4. Prevent your platelets from clumping;
5. Improve your arterial flexibility;
6. Increase your lifespan.

One large study from Europe reported that a higher intake of polyphenols—particularly grapes, nuts and flax—was associated with a longer lifespan.

Still need more proof? In over 34,000 post-menopausal women, eating bran, apples, pears, grapefruit, strawberries, red wine and chocolate was associated with a lower risk of heart disease and all-cause deaths.

Whole foods with polyphenols are great for you. That is not B.S.

More information is available in an article I wrote entitled "10 Best Polyphenol-Rich Superfoods + Why You Should Be Eating Them" at www.mindbodygreen.com/0-17145/10-best-polyphenol-rich-superfoods-why-you-should-be-eating-them.html.

Lesson: Meat and Type 2 Diabetes – Fact or B.S.?

Meat has to be OK, right? It cannot be B.S. if I see my doctor out at a party eating a steak? Well, maybe your doctor, brother-in-law or boss should read the latest science connecting eating meat and the risk of type 2 diabetes, a major cause of illness and death.

Let's take a No B.S. look at this:
- In 1985, the Adventist Mortality Study analyzed the risk of diabetes in 25,000 vegetarians and meat eaters and found that women who ate red meat had an increased risk of developing diabetes by 40 percent while men who ate red meat increased their risk by 80 percent.
- In 1999, the Adventist Health Study looked at 34,000 Seventh-day Adventists and found that women who ate meat increased their risk of developing diabetes by 93 percent; for men the figure was 97 percent.
- In 2009, the Adventist Health-2 Study evaluated 61,000 people and found that meat eaters were twice as likely to develop diabetes as those whose diets were totally plant-based.
- In the Nurses Health Study I and II involving 195,000 participants, diabetes risk went up with the number of times fish was consumed weekly, perhaps due to the pollutants in fish.

Diet is a personal decision, but in the midst of an epidemic of type 2 diabetes soon to impact 100 million Americans (and many more worldwide), avoiding diabetes is critical.

Eating meat can now be added to physical inactivity, obesity, ingesting excessive quantities of added dietary sugars and polycystic ovarian syndrome (PCOS) as a risk factor for developing type 2 diabetes.

To read more, see my article entitled "Could Eating Meat Give You Diabetes? A Cardiologist Explains" at www.mindbodygreen.com/0-14908/could-eating-meat-give-you-diabetes-a-cardiologist-explains.html.

Lesson: Eat and Live a Heart Attack-Free Life

Several recently completed studies demonstrate how easily we can protect ourselves against heart attacks.

Two great studies and what they mean for you:

1. The MORGEN Study.
    *   Researchers in the Netherlands studied almost 18,000 men and women without heart disease, following them for up to 14 years.
    *   More than 600 of the group had heart attacks, including deaths.
    *   The study found that if people followed these four steps they were able to lower their risk of heart attacks by 67 percent:

        1. Averaging 30 minutes a day of physical activity improved health outcomes;
        2. Eating a healthy diet in the Mediterranean style, rich in fruits, vegetables and whole grains;
        3. Not smoking;
        4. Enjoying more than one alcoholic beverage a month.
        5. People who added a fifth health habit—sleeping seven or more hours a night on average—lowered their risk of heart attacks by 83 percent compared to those not following these steps.

2. The Karolinska Study.
    *   Scientists in Sweden studied over 20,000 men who were free of heart disease by following them for 11 years.
    *   They found that certain habits lowered the risk of heart attacks, including:

        1. A diet rich in fruits, vegetables, legumes, nuts, whole grains and reduced fat;
        2. Not smoking;
        3. Moderate daily alcohol consumption;
        4. Thin waistlines;
        5. More than 40 minutes of daily physical activity.

Lesson: Eat and Live a Heart Attack-Free Life *(Cont'd)*

So it's as easy as simply sticking to habits and not having a heart attack.

You can read more details in my article entitled "Simple Lifestyle Changes You Can Make To Avoid A Heart Attack" at www.mindbodygreen.com/0-16072/simple-lifestyle-changes-you-can-make-to-avoid-a-heart-attack.html.

Lesson: What You Should Know About Finland

What was Finland's problem? In the early 1970s, young men in Finland were dying from heart attacks at the highest rates in the industrialized world. Every family knew the pain of watching a young and fit man die prematurely.

In 1972, the Finnish government launched the North Karelia Project with the goal of lowering the quantity and type of fats eaten and to decrease smoking rates. Residents were asked to switch from butter to vegetable oil-based margarine and replace whole milk with low-fat milk.

Did the residents respond? They sure did.

The rate of using butter on bread fell from 90 percent to less than five percent. And one third of the population began to drink skim or one percent milk, up from zero at the outset. Overall dietary fat intake dropped and saturated fats fell to 16 percent of calories.

What were the results? The change in the rate of those dying at a young age was stunning. In North Karelia, overall death of men between the ages of 35 and 64 years dropped by 62 percent; heart attack deaths fell by 85 percent; and deaths from all types of cancer dropped by 65 percent, including a decrease in lung cancer by 80 percent.

For the entire Finnish nation, the chance of dying from a heart attack during working years was reduced by a whopping 80 percent! When researchers looked at what caused the dramatic improvements in health, they found that the most powerful factor was the reduction in saturated fat from animal sources.

As a cardiologist with decades of experience, my advice to you is this: If anyone recommends you eat a diet high in animal fats, ask them if they have any long-term data on preventing heart disease, the number one killer in the world. Tell them about the miracle in Finland that happened when they dropped butter from their diet.

If you want to read more, you can find my article entitled "Why You Should Eat More Plants & Fewer Animals (Lessons From Finland)" at www.mindbodygreen.com/0-13289/why-you-should-eat-more-plants-fewer-animals-lessons-from-finland.html.

Lesson: New No B.S. Ways Red Meat May Be a Danger to Your Health

If we aren't allowing science to guide us in our health decisions, then we are probably basing those decisions on some B.S. opinion. So let's review some new data.

Over 121,000 doctors and nurses provided dietary histories for patients they followed up to 28 years. The relationship between eating red meat and early death established that each daily single serving increase of red meat upped the risk of dying from any cause.

Processed meats, such as bologna and hot dogs, posed more risk than unprocessed red meat. The risk for cancer followed the same ugly trend.

European researchers followed 448,000 men and women for years. Their findings were that red meat, particularly processed red meat, was associated with early death.

They estimated that three percent of all deaths would be avoided if we kept pepperoni, salami, hot dogs and other processed meats to less than 20 grams a day.

How about a whole new pathway implicating meat and eggs in heart disease?

Researchers at the Cleveland Clinic published data finding that red meat is high in the chemical carnitine (remember: carne equals meat) and egg yolks are very high in another chemical choline, a point I'll get to shortly.

So what? Intestinal bacterial in meat eaters converts carnitine into a chemical called TMAO.

TMAO then gets into the bloodstream and directly adds plaque to arteries.

If you don't eat meat and eggs regularly, you don't make TMAO— and your arteries are healthier.

That is the science. What we do with it is personal. But it is B.S. to say that eating large amounts of animal-based foods, as some Paleo caveman diet advocates argue, is healthy for us.

TMAO is dangerous. We have more to learn, such as the benefits of choline for the brain, but for now, caution is advised.

More details are in my article entitled "Is Eating Red Meat Dangerous? A Cardiologist Explains" at www.mindbodygreen.com/0-8759/is-eating-red-meat-dangerous-a-cardiologist-explains.html.

Lesson: Dietary Salt Causes Disease – No B.S., But is Often Hidden

Refined salt is easy to spot and control in a shaker or on a chip, but it's not so easy to identify in many processed foods, restaurant items or kitchen staples.

If you're looking to reduce your sodium intake to improve your health (current guidelines suggest 1,500 to 2,300 milligrams of sodium daily), as is recommended in the popular DASH diet (Dietary Approaches to Stop Hypertension), then you might want to keep an eye on the following five items:

1. Processed red meats. Packaged ham, bacon, sausage, turkey and many deli meats are high in sodium, which is added to preserve the meat from spoilage. A serving may have over half the day's recommended sodium load.
2. Poultry. Sodium is often injected into poultry during processing. Read labels when buying chicken in the grocery store as this can help you make better choices.
3. Soup. Many canned chicken noodle soups also have about 1,000 mg of sodium. If you want soup, make it yourself or else carefully read the label before buying. Opt for the one with the least amount of sodium.
4. Pizza. The dough and cheese of a typical slice have over a third of the day's recommended sodium load. Ask questions, cut back or skip the cheese in favor of more veggies. Better yet, make your own.
5. Bread and rolls. Store-bought bread is a hidden source of refined salt. By some estimates, sodium from bread is the number one source of salt in the average diet. Again, be sure to read labels, selecting brands with lower amounts of sodium.

For more details my article entitled "6 Foods That Have WAY Too Much Sodium" is at www.mindbodygreen.com/0-14214/6-foods-that-have-way-too-much-sodium.html.

Lesson: Eggs Are Healthy – Fact or B.S.?

In 2011, the US Department of Agriculture published the *Dietary Guidelines for Americans* and included eggs among the foods to reduce.

Eating up to one egg a day (including those found in breads and baked goods) was considered acceptable for healthy folks, but in patients with heart issues or diabetes, the recommendation was to eat less than 0.4 ounces a day—that's about a quarter of an egg. Not a glowing endorsement. Also, I imagine it's hard to scramble a quarter of an egg!

A team of medical researchers decided to investigate eggs. Using ultrasound, they looked at the amount of plaque found in carotid arteries in the necks of over 1,000 people. Patients who ate more than three eggs a week had increased plaque compared to those who ate two or less eggs a week, even after other risks like smoking were factored in.

Chinese researchers reviewed 17 studies on eggs and health. They found no overall relationship between egg consumption and heart disease. However, among people with diabetes, those whose egg intake was highest had 1.5 times the risk of heart disease compared to those who ate the fewest eggs.

Finally, the choline in eggs has made headlines around the world. Eating two hard-boiled eggs led to a rise in TMAO in the blood within minutes, just as eating red meat did.

TMAO promotes arteries getting clogged up!

If you do eat eggs, concentrate on the egg whites, free of cholesterol and saturated fat.

For more details, check out my article entitled "Are Eggs Healthy Or Not? A Cardiologist Explains" at www.mindbodygreen.com/0-9205/are-eggs-healthy-or-not-a-cardiologist-explains.html.

Lesson: Spices Can Turbo-Charge Your Health

One of the simplest ways to power your No B.S. Diet is to use spices (free of processed salt, of course).

How can spices help?

- Apple Pie Spice. This powerhouse mixture usually has cinnamon, cloves, allspice and nutmeg. By sprinkling this tasty and sugar-free mix on your food and drinks, you can boost the antioxidant level of meals substantially. Antioxidants work to reverse the "rusting" and aging effects of stress and toxins on your arteries and other organs.
- In addition to cloves, cinnamon helps balance your blood sugar and decreases bad cholesterol; allspice lowers blood pressure and may relieve menopause symptoms; and nutmeg may prevent wrinkles, lower cholesterol, treat depression and improve memory.
- Italian Seasoning Mix. The ingredients of these green flake mixtures may include marjoram, thyme, basil, rosemary and sage. Italian mixtures fare very well in antioxidant activity. For example, rosemary has been known since the time of Shakespeare to improve memory. Adding this mixture to grilled foods may lessen the production of chemicals that promote aging and cancer.
- Curry Powder. An infinite number of blends exist for this potent Indian mix. The bottle in my kitchen contains coriander, cumin, turmeric, chili pepper, ginger, cardamom, mustard, cloves, nutmeg, black pepper and saffron. Thousands of research studies done on animals and humans show health benefits from turmeric and curcumin in many medical illnesses ranging from heart disease, diabetes, Alzheimer's disease and cancer.

You can read more about the benefits of spices in my article entitled "3 Spice Bottles That Protect Your Heart And Reduce Inflammation" at www.mindbodygreen.com/0-7649/3-spice-bottles-that-protect-your-heart-and-reduce-inflammation.html.

Lesson: The No B.S. Diet Can Reverse Diseases

Can you really reverse disease conditions and reduce or eliminate medications with plant-based diets? Let's hear from four of my friends who decided to eat totally plant based and find out whether or not it is B.S.

- Allan, Podiatrist. When he started, he carried 274 pounds on his 5'7" frame, he was taking medications and he would become short of breath when climbing stairs.
- Allan reported: "It's been 13 months since that start date. My waist went from a 44 to 34, my neck went from 18.5 to 17 inches and I lost 76 pounds. My blood pressure normalized and my cholesterol numbers got into a very healthy range. I stopped taking the cholesterol medicine."

- Neal, Musician. Following heart bypass surgery, he spent years taking medications for high blood pressure and high cholesterol as well as insulin for type 2 diabetes. He agreed to try a whole-foods, plant-based diet.
- Neal said: "In a little over two months, my blood sugar remained in the 80s to 90s range, and I was able to discontinue my insulin. Blood work at my doctor's office also indicated my total cholesterol had dropped over 100 points and my triglycerides level was cut in half!"

- Marc, Former Football Star. Marc had a strong family history of diabetes and developed it himself.
- Marc said that in late 2011, "My in-laws gave my wife, Kim, and myself a copy of *Forks Over Knives*. In less than two months I was off of all my medications. It's been almost three years since I began my new lifestyle, and I'm proud to say that as of my last reading, I am no longer diabetic."

Lesson: The No B.S. Diet Can Reverse Diseases *(Cont'd)*

- <u>Paul, Consultant</u>. Paul traveled to the Cleveland Clinic in early 2013 with chest pains, only to find out he had one fully blocked artery and two mostly blocked arteries.
- Paul said: "I switched to plant-based nutrition. For nearly two years I've learned how to cook meals with fruits, vegetables, legumes and whole grains without added oils. I've lost 45 pounds and lowered my cholesterol from 298 to 132."

<u>Disease reversal and elimination of medications can and does happen for many people who make the necessary changes—and take action. That is not B.S.</u>

For more details, my article entitled "Before & After: Plant-Based Diet Success Stories" is at <u>www.mindbodygreen.com/0-17625/before-after-plant-based-diet-success-stories.html</u>.

Lesson: How You Prepare Food Is No B.S. Decision

An important, but overlooked component of nutrition is how you cook your food.

First you need to know about modified proteins and fats called *advanced glycation end products* (commonly referred to as AGEs). Higher levels of AGEs contribute to diabetes mellitus, and they are known to fire up inflammation leading to heart disease, obesity and arthritis.

Frying and grilling foods (particularly dry grilling like BBQing), are among the highest sources of AGEs in our diet.

For example, French fries from fast food chains have nearly 90 times the amount of AGEs of a boiled potato.

Grilled or broiled chicken and chicken nuggets have up to 10 times the amount of AGEs of boiled chicken.

Even a fried egg has 50 times the AGE level of a boiled egg.

Butter and cheeses are naturally high in AGE content and can have three times the amount of a grilled piece of meat.

Vegetables are naturally low in AGEs and their high water content protects them from AGE production when heated.

What Can We Do to Avoid AGEing?

Healthy vegetarian and vegan diets are naturally low in AGEs and may be responsible for the longer lifespan of vegetarians and vegans.

However, here are some grilling tips:
- Avoid charred and blackened meats. This is wise because of the high AGE content and a reported link to pancreatic cancer.
- If you're going to grill, marinate meat before and during cooking. Moistened meats produce half of the AGEs of dry meats. Lemon juice and vinegar combinations are particularly good marinades.
- Cook for shorter times at lower heat. Avoid the high flames from extra lighter fluids and dripping fats.
- Clean your grill. Keep the grill clean of old burnt residues. Or grill on tin foil to help avoid charring.
- Consider steaming, poaching or boiling your foods. Avoid the grill entirely.

Lesson: How You Prepare Food Is No B.S. Decision *(Cont'd)*

Read more details about avoiding AGEs in my article entitled "Why You Should Think Twice About That BBQ: A Cardiologist Explains" at www.mindbodygreen.com/0-10024/why-you-should-think-twice-about-that-bbq-a-cardiologist-explains.html.

Lesson: All the Info, None of The B.S., to Learn More About Eating Plants

By now you've gotten the message: eat more fruits and vegetables and less animal products if you want the health, not the B.S.

Here are some resources to help you get energized for success.

- Kaiser Permanente. The largest managed care organization in the USA provides strong medical support for a whole-foods, plant-based diet, as well as pages of practical tips in their downloadable resources.
- Physicians Committee for Responsible Medicine (PCRM). This organization, led by Dr. Neal Barnard, maintains high standards and does original research. For example, PCRM has found evidence that diabetes mellitus in adults can be treated and reversed with plant-based diets. Their Vegetarian Starter Kit is an excellent tool.
- PCRM offers a 21-Day Vegan Kickstart program, beginning on the first of every month and is available in several languages. It's free and includes celebrity tips, meal plans, webcasts, restaurant guides, daily messages and a community forum. I highly recommend signing up.
- *Forks Over Knives*. I ask all of my patients to watch this documentary with their families. It has the biggest impact on deciding to eat a healthier diet than any other resource I've found. The film's website provides a guide to eating that is another great resource.
- Animals Deserve Absolute Protection Today and Tomorrow (ADAPTT). This organization's website, www.adaptt.org, was created by animal liberation activist Gary Yourofsky and features his viral 70-minute speech making the case for a vegan diet. The site has great resources for changing to plant-based nutrition.

Lesson: All the Info, None of The B.S., to Learn More About Eating
Plants *(Cont'd)*

The resources above can benefit anyone hoping to improve health,
reverse disease or manage weight. Eating a plant-based diet reduces
damage to the planet and to animals while making you healthier. It's a
win-win-win we can all embrace.

You can learn more by reading my article entitled "Everything
You Need To Know To Start A Plant-Based Diet" at
www.mindbodygreen.com/0-14670/everything-you-need-to-know-to-
start-a-plant-based-diet.html.

If You Only Have 10 Minutes Again: The Results of the No B.S. Diet

Leading Causes of Death that Plant-Based Diets Reverse and Prevent

- Heart disease
- Cancer
- Chronic lung disease
- Brain diseases like stroke
- Alzheimer's dementia
- Diabetes Mellitus
- Pneumonia and influenza
- Kidney disease

The No B.S. Secret

Eighty percent of all deaths from the above eight causes not related to accidents or suicide revolve around three habits:
- Whether we smoke;
- Whether we eat well (defined as fruits, vegetables, whole grains and legumes);
- Whether we move well (walking and fitness).

Part II. What Do We Die of? What Can We Do Without the B.S.?

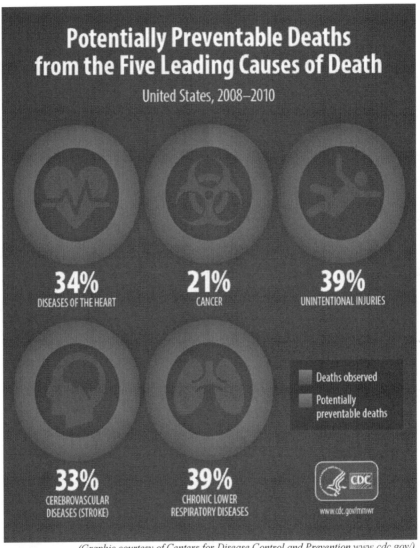

(Graphic courtesy of Centers for Disease Control and Prevention www.cdc.gov/)

Heart Disease and Nutrition – So Much B.S, But So Much Data

Three statements to take to heart:

1. "Vegetarian diets are associated with lower all-cause mortality and with some reductions in cause-specific mortality. Results appeared to be more robust in males. These favorable associations should be considered carefully by those offering dietary guidance," according to *The Journal of the American Medical Association (JAMA) Internal Medicine*.

2. "More regression of coronary atherosclerosis occurred after five years than after one year in the experimental group [10 percent fat whole foods vegetarian diet, aerobic exercise, stress management training, smoking cessation, group psychosocial support]. In contrast, in the control group, coronary atherosclerosis continued to progress and more than twice as many cardiac events occurred," per *JAMA*.

3. "Plant-based nutrition has the potential for a large effect on the CVD epidemic," says the *Journal of Family Practice*.

The No B.S. Takeaway: Most cases of heart disease are "foodborne" illnesses that can be prevented and even reversed by plant-based diets.

Low fat vegan diets studied by Drs. Ornish and Esselstyn have improved symptoms within three weeks and reversed proven heart disease. Eat your damn vegetables and fruits every damn day every meal and snack. Got it?

Cancer and Diet: Is There No B.S. Science?

Four powerful statements relating cancer and diet:

1. "The incidence of all cancers combined was lower among vegetarians than among meat eaters," per the results from the European Prospective Investigation into Cancer and Nutrition.

2. "The consumption of poultry was related to an increased risk of B-cell lymphomas," according to the *International Journal of Cancer*.

3. "Intensive lifestyle changes (low fat vegetarian diet) may affect the progression of early, low grade prostate cancer in men," according to the *Journal of Urology*.

4. "Adherence to a plant-based diet that limits red meat intake may be associated with reduced risk of breast cancer, particularly in postmenopausal women," per the *American Journal of Clinical Nutrition*.

The International Agency for Research on Cancer (IARC) of the World Health Organization announced in October 2015 that processed red meats like bacon, ham, hot dogs and salami had enough evidence linked to cancer to be classified as Class I carcinogens—the same as cigarettes! The rest of the meat world was classified as 2A, on par with dangerous pesticides in terms of cancer risk.

The No B.S. Takeaway: Some cancers occur much less frequently with plant-based diets (fruits, vegetables, beans, nuts and seeds). Established cancer, particularly prostate, responds favorably to plant-based diets.

Meat and particularly processed meats like hot dogs, bologna and sausage are linked to higher cancer rates. Don't eat them if you want to meet your grandchildren or see them grow up. You do not need cow's milk unless you are a cow. Try almond, rice, soy, hemp or oat milk, yogurts, faux cheeses or ice cream.

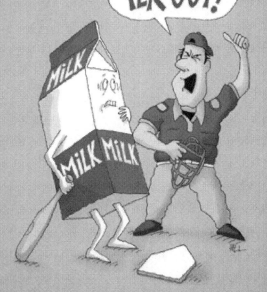

(Graphic courtesy of Physicians Committee for Responsible Medicine www.pcrm.org)

Chronic Lung Disease: COPD, Emphysema, Bronchitis and No B.S.
Foods

Your lungs and your diet are connected!

1. "Higher antioxidant food intake (fresh fruit and vegetables) may be associated with improvement in lung function, and in this respect, dietary interventions might be considered in COPD," according to the *European Respiratory Journal*.

2. "A high fat diet may contribute to chronic inflammatory disease of the airway and lung," according to the *European Journal of Applied Physiology*.

The No B.S. Takeaway: Processed junk foods increase inflammation in the lungs. Plant-based choices reduce inflammation, allowing lung disease to improve. If you are eating fast food, you are inviting fast death and illness.

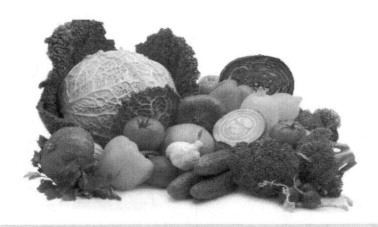

Diet For COPD

Stroke: Prevention by Diet

Preventing a stroke is within your control.

1. "A healthy lifestyle (five or more servings per day of fruits and vegetables and less than 30 grams per day of processed meat) is associated with a substantially reduced risk of stroke in men at higher risk of stroke," according to an article in *Neurology*.

2. "These findings indicate that intake of dietary fiber, especially fruit and vegetable fibers, is inversely associated with risk of stroke," per an article in the *Journal of Nutrition*.

The No B.S. Takeaway: Many cases of stroke are related to bad arteries, high blood pressure, obesity and diabetes. Plant-based diets rich in fiber can reduce stroke deaths. If you eat crap, you will have a crap brain.

Food sources of fiber include whole wheat, bran, fresh or dried fruits, and vegetables

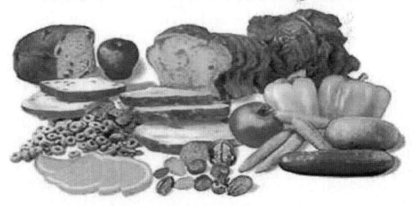

(Graphic courtesy of DianeSays.com www.dianesays.com/)

Alzheimer's Dementia: No B.S. Data Points to Ponder

Your diet does matter when it comes to having control over memory loss and your intellectual abilities.

1. "The matched subjects who ate meat (including poultry and fish) were more than twice as likely to become demented as their vegetarian counterparts," according to the preliminary findings from the Adventist Health Study.

2. "Several lines of evidence provide support for the hypothesis that high saturated or trans fatty acids increase the risk of dementia," per the journal *Neurobiology of Aging*.

3. The seven guidelines to reduce risk of Alzheimer's disease are:
   - Minimize your intake of saturated fats and trans fats. Saturated fat is found primarily in dairy products, meats and certain oils (coconut and palm oils).
   - Eat plant-based foods. Vegetables, legumes (beans, peas and lentils), fruits and whole grains should replace meats and dairy products as primary staples of the diet.
   - Consume 15 milligrams of vitamin E from foods each day. Healthful food sources of vitamin E include seeds, nuts, green leafy vegetables and whole grains.
   - Take a B12 supplement.
   - Avoid vitamins with iron and copper.
   - Choose aluminum-free products like deodorants.
   - Exercise for 120 minutes each week. Include aerobic exercise in your routine, equivalent to 40 minutes of brisk walking, three times per week.

Adapted from "Dietary Guidelines for Alzheimer's Prevention" by The Physicians Committee for Responsible Medicine. www.pcrm.org/health/reports/dietary-guidelines-for-alzheimers-prevention.

Alzheimer's Dementia: No B.S. Data Points to Ponder

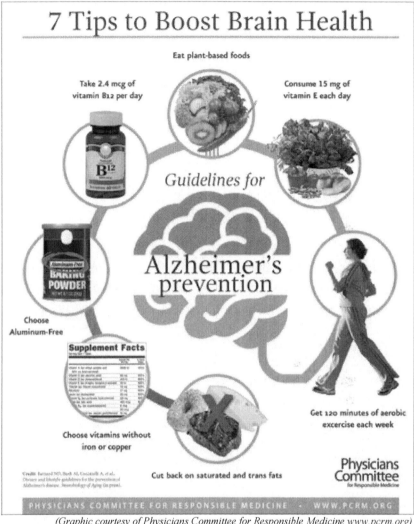

(Graphic courtesy of Physicians Committee for Responsible Medicine www.pcrm.org)

Diabetes Mellitus: The No B.S. Science to Manage and Reverse This Killer

A diagnosis of diabetes is not permanent!

1. "Cases of diabetes developed in 0.54% of vegans and 2.12% of non-vegetarians. Vegetarian diets were associated with a substantial and independent reduction in diabetes," per *Nutrition, Metabolism and Cardiovascular Diseases.*

2. "Low-fat plant-based nutrition improves control of weight, glycemia and heart risk. Vegetarian and vegan diets present potential advantages in managing type 2 diabetes," according to *Current Diabetes Reports.*

The No B.S. Takeaway for diabetes: type 2 (adult-onset) diabetes is related to processed diets heavy in animal products that pack muscles with fat and render them resistant to insulin. Reversal of diabetes by shifting to a low-fat, plant-based diet is a very successful approach in as little as two weeks. Eat your damn vegetables. Every day.

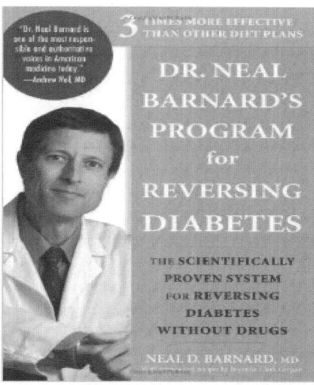

(Graphic courtesy of Neal D. Barnard, MD www.pcrm.org)

Pneumonia: Immune Boosting by Nutrition is No B.S.

Easily enhance your health.

1. "Increased fruit and vegetable consumption may improve vaccination response in older people, linking an achievable dietary goal to a potential improvement in immune function," according to *Proceedings of the Nutrition Society*.

2. "Embracing a cuisine rich in spice, as well as in fruit and vegetables, may further enhance the chemo-preventive capacity of one's diet," according to the *American Journal of Clinical Nutrition*.

The No B.S. Takeaway: Better nutrition can lead to better immune function. Plant-based diets provide necessary vitamins, minerals and antioxidants. Add spices every day.

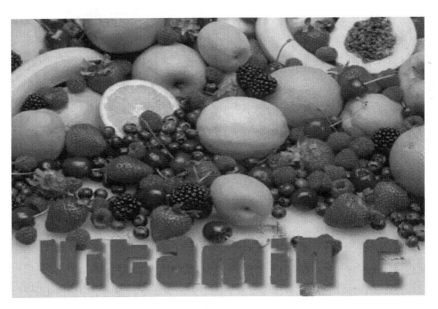

Kidney Disease: Are Meat Calories or Plant Calories Best?

Your kidneys need your attention.

1. "Higher dietary intake of animal fat and two or more servings per week of red meat may increase risk for microalbuminuria (kidney damage)," according to the *Clinical Journal of the American Society of Nephrology.*

2. "Of the studied parameters, it was found that urine protein was significantly different in vegans and controls. Vegans had a significantly lower urine protein level," according to the journal, *Renal Failure.*

The No B.S. Takeaway: Kidney function may be harmed by animal products and protected by plant-based diets. Protect your kidney beans by eating kidney beans. Every day.

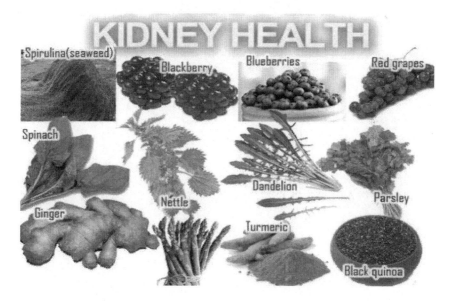

Part III: The No B.S. Diet Plate

I always lecture groups showing this healthy eating plate from the Harvard School of Public Health. Study it and you will have a great guide to health and disease prevention and reversal. It is a clean eating program on one page.

I hope it becomes your plate as of today.

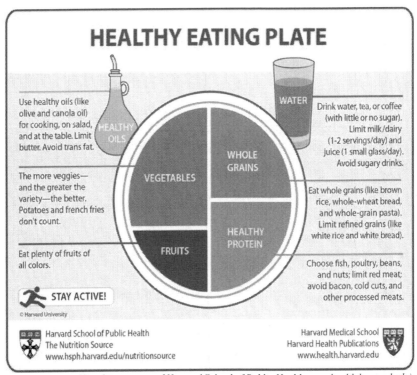

(Graphic courtesy of Harvard School of Public Health www.health.harvard.edu)

The No B.S. Diet Rules

- <u>Eat whole fruit</u> not fruit juice.

- <u>Eat steel-cut (not packaged) oatmeal</u> and no Frosted Flakes!

- <u>Eat broccoli</u> not French fries—and don't whine about it.

- <u>Drink water</u> not soda or energy drinks with sugar.

- <u>Add plain nuts</u> not potato chips as a snack at work.

- <u>Eat more than five servings of fruits and veggies a day</u>.

- <u>Donuts will make you impotent</u>—think about that.

- <u>If you can't pronounce the ingredient list, skip it</u>. A banana comes with no list.

- <u>If it says natural or healthy, it probably isn't!</u>

- <u>Spices heal</u>; added sugar causes illness.

- <u>A sandwich on white bread, without lettuce and tomato, is a waste of time!</u>

- <u>Food companies in general couldn't care less about your health.</u>

- <u>Food is information, good or bad</u>. Every bite you make.

Taking the Next Steps to Launching the No B.S. Diet

I have laid out the resources you need to start learning more about how to implement the No B.S. Diet in an article I wrote entitled "Everything You Need to Know To Start A Plant-Based Diet" at www.mindbodygreen.com/0-14670/everything-you-need-to-know-to-start-a-plant-based-diet.html.

Another great resource I use every day in my clinic is the website www.21daykickstart.org. I encourage you to sign up and take a free, three-week plunge into eating healthy. This resource will provide you with the tools and motivation to start a new life plan if you care about your health.

Warning! You may encounter one potential side effect: you might feel better, lose weight and require less medication!

For more practical tips, read "The Heart Doctor's Wife 3 Day Eating Plan" prepared by Karen Kahn, RN, BSN. Karen is a licensed Nurse, Certified Nutritionist and holistic coach. You will find practical, tasty and easy to prepare recipes.

Further information and programs for health are available for free at drjoelkahn.com and kahnlongevitycenter.com.

BIBLIOGRAPHY

Heart Disease and Nutrition: So Much B.S., But So Much Data

Orlich, MJ, PN Singh, J. Sabaté, K Jaceldo-Siegl, J Fan, S Knutsen, WL Beeson and GE Fraser. "Vegetarian Dietary Patterns and Mortality in Adventist Health Study 2." http://www.ncbi.nlm.nih.gov/pubmed/23836264. JAMA Intern Med. 2013 Jul 8;173(13):1230-8. Web. 9 Nov. 2015.

Ornish D, LW Scherwitz, JH Billings, SE Brown, KL Gould, TA Merritt, S Sparler, WT Armstrong, TA Ports, RL Kirkeeide, C Hogeboom and RJ Brand. "Intensive lifestyle changes for reversal of coronary heart disease." http://www.ncbi.nlm.nih.gov/pubmed/9863851. JAMA. 1998 Dec 16;280(23):2001-7. Erratum in JAMA 1999 Apr 21;281(15):1380. Web. 9 Nov. 2015.

CB Esselstyn Jr, G Gendy, J Doyle, M Golubic and MF Roizen. "A way to reverse CAD?" http://www.ncbi.nlm.nih.gov/pubmed/25198208. J Fam Practice 2014 Jul;63(7):356-364b. Web. 9 Nov. 2015.

Cancer and Diet: Is There No B.S. Science?

Key, TJ, PN Appleby, EA Spencer, RC Travis, AW Roddam and NE Allen. "Cancer incidence in vegetarians: results from the European Prospective Investigation into Cancer and Nutrition. (EPIC-Oxford)." http://ajcn.nutrition.org/content/89/5/1620S.abstract. Am J Clin Nutr vol. 89 no. 5 1620S-1626S. Web. 9 Nov. 2015.

Rohrmann, S, J Linseisen, MU Jakobsen, K Overvad, O Raaschou-Nielsen, A Tjonneland, MC Boutron-Ruault, R Kaaks, N Becker, M Bergmann, H Boeing, KT Khaw, NJ Wareham, TJ Key, R Travis, V Benetou, A Naska, A Trichopoulou, V Pala, R Tumino, G Masala, A Mattiello, M Brustad, E Lund, G Skeie, HB Bueno-de-Mesquita, PH Peeters, RC Vermeulen, P Jakszyn, M Dorronsoro, A Barricarte, MJ Tormo, E Molina, M Argüelles, B Melin, U Ericson, J Manjer, S Rinaldi, N Slimani, P Boffetta, AC Vergnaud, A Khan, T Norat and P Vineis. "Consumption of meat and dairy and lymphoma risk in the European Prospective Investigation into Cancer and Nutrition." http://www.ncbi.nlm.nih.gov/pubmed/20473877. Int J Cancer. 2011 Feb 1;128(3):623-34. doi: 10.1002/ijc.25387. Web. 9 Nov. 2015.

Ornish, D, G Weidner, WR Fair, R Marlin, EB Pettengill, CJ Raisin, S Dunn-Emke, L Crutchfield, FN Jacobs, RJ Barnard, WJ Aronson, P McCormac, DJ McKnight, JD Fein, AM Dnistrian, J Weinstein, TH Ngo, NR Mendell and PR Carroll. "Intensive lifestyle changes may affect the progression of prostate cancer." http://www.ncbi.nlm.nih.gov/pubmed/16094059. J Urol. 2005 Sep;174(3):1065-9; discussion 1069-70. Web. 9 Nov. 2015.

Catsburg, C, RS Kim, VA Kirsh, CL Soskolne, N Kreiger and TE Rohan. "Dietary patterns and breast cancer risk: a study in 2 cohorts." http://www.ncbi.nlm.nih.gov/pubmed/25833979. Am J Clin Nutr. 2015 Apr;101(4):817-23. doi: 10.3945/ajcn.114.097659. Epub 2015 Feb 11. Web. 9 Nov. 2015.

Chronic Lung Disease: COPD, Emphysema, Bronchitis and No B.S. Foods

Keranis, E, D Makris, P Rodopoulou, H Martinou, G Papamakarios, Z Daniil, E Zintzaras, and KI Gourgoulianis. "Impact of dietary shift to higher-antioxidant foods in COPD: a randomised trial." http://www.ncbi.nlm.nih.gov/pubmed/20150206. Eur Respir J. 2010 Oct;36(4):774-80. doi: 10.1183/09031936.00113809. Epub 2010 Feb 11. Web. 9 Nov. 2015.

Rosenkranz, SK, DK Townsend, SE Steffens, and CA Harms. "Effects of a high-fat meal on pulmonary function in healthy subjects." http://www.ncbi.nlm.nih.gov/pubmed/20165863. Eur J Appl Physiol. 2010 Jun;109(3):499-506. doi: 10.1007/s00421-010-1390-1. Epub 2010 Feb 18. Web. 9 Nov. 2015.

Stroke: Prevention by Diet

Larsson, SC, A Åkesson and A Wolk. "Primary prevention of stroke by a healthy lifestyle in a high-risk group." http://www.ncbi.nlm.nih.gov/pubmed/25934859. Epub 2015 May 1. Web. 9 Nov. 2015.

Larsson, SC and A Wolk. "Dietary fiber intake is inversely associated with stroke incidence in healthy Swedish adults." http://www.ncbi.nlm.nih.gov/pubmed/25411032. J Nutr. 2014 Dec;144(12):1952-5. doi: 10.3945/jn.114.200634. Epub 2014 Sep 24. Web 9 Nov. 2015.

Alzheimer's Dementia: No B.S. Data Points to Ponder

Giem, P, WL Beeson, and GE Fraser. "The incidence of dementia and intake of animal products: preliminary findings from the Adventist Health Study." http://www.ncbi.nlm.nih.gov/pubmed/8327020. Neuroepidemiology 1993:12;28-36. Web 9 Nov. 2015.

Morris, MC and CC Tangney. "Dietary fat composition and dementia risk." http://www.ncbi.nlm.nih.gov/pubmed/24970568. Neurobiol Aging. 2014 Sep;35 Suppl 2:S59-64. doi:10.1016/j.neurobiolaging.2014.03.038. Epub 2014 May 15. Web 9 Nov. 2015.

Diabetes Mellitus: The No B.S. Science to Manage and Reverse This Killer

Tonstad S, K Stewart, K Oda, M Batech, RP Herring and GE Fraser. "Vegetarian diets and incidence of diabetes in the Adventist Health Study-2." http://www.ncbi.nlm.nih.gov/pubmed/21983060. Nutr Metab Cardiovasc Dis. 2013 Apr;23(4):292-9. doi:10.1016/j.numecd.2011.07.004. Epub 2011 Oct 7. Web. 9 Nov. 2015.

Trapp, CB and ND Barnard. "Usefulness of Vegetarian and Vegan Diets for Treating Type 2 Diabetes." Current Diabetes Reports. April 2010, Volume 10, Issue 2, pp 152-158. First online: 09 March 2010

Pneumonia: Immune Boosting by Nutrition is No B.S.

Edgar, JD, A Gibson, CE Neville, SECM Gilchrist, MC Mckinley, CC Patterson, IS Young and JV Woodside. "Increased fruit and vegetable consumption improves antibody response to vaccination in older people: the ADIT study." http://journals.cambridge.org/action/displayAbstract?fromPage=online&aid=7791675&fileId=S0029665110000273. Proceedings of the Nutrition Society 2010 69:E238. Web. 9 Nov. 2015.

Lampe, JW. "Spicing up a vegetarian diet: chemopreventive effects of phytochemicals." http://www.ncbi.nlm.nih.gov/pubmed/12936952. Am J Clin Nutr. 2003 Sep;78(3 Suppl):579S-583S. Web. 9 Nov. 2015.

Kidney Disease: Are Meat Calories or Plant Calories Best?

Lin, J, FB Hu and GC Curhan. "Associations of Diet with Albuminuria and Kidney Function Decline." http://www.ncbi.nlm.nih.gov/pmc/articles/PMC2863979. Clin J Am Soc Nephrol. 2010 May; 5(5): 836–843. doi: 10.2215/CJN.08001109. PMCID: PMC2863979. Web. 9 Nov. 2015.

Wiwanitkit, V. "Renal function parameters of Thai vegans compared with non-vegans." http://www.ncbi.nlm.nih.gov/pubmed/17365939. Ren Fail. 2007;29(2):219-20. Web. 9 Nov. 2015

Made in the USA
Middletown, DE
14 January 2018